THE NEW LYMPHEDEMA AND LIPEDEMA DIET

Savor Over 1500 Days of Nourishing Recipes for Losing Weight, Reducing Swelling, Improving Metabolic Health and Preventing Complications

Dr. Anna Fennell

COPYRIGHT

Copyright © 2024 by Dr. Anna Fennell

TABLE OF CONTENTS

JUST ONE FINAL THING TO ADDRESS BEFORE YOU GO!

INTRODUCTION

Lipoedema (lip-o-dee-muh) is a chronic disorder of fat metabolism and distribution which usually manifests as a disproportionate amount of fat being stored in the lower half of the body. Whilst lipoedema may affect both men and women, it's most commonly seen in women. Lipoedema sufferers will present with a disproportionate amount of fat stored in the outer thighs, inner thighs, lower legs and ankles, and sometimes the upper arms. In severe cases, the fatty collections can be quite disfiguring, leading to problems with joints and mobility. The cause of lipoedema is unknown however many doctors believe it's linked to hormones, particularly in women as many symptoms develop or worsen during times of extreme hormonal changes such as puberty, pregnancy, or menopause. Those suffering from lipoedema experience hormonal disturbances, frequent bruising of the skin, and develop tissue that feels rubbery to touch. Lipoedema is a progressive disease and will worsen with age. Some studies have shown that lipoedema may run in families.

CHAPTER ONE

WHAT IS LYMPHEDEMA?

Lymphedema manifests as the swelling of one or more extremities due to a disruption in the flow of the lymphatic system. The lymphatic system constitutes a complex network of specialized vessels, known as lymph vessels, distributed throughout the body. Its primary function is to collect excess lymph fluid containing proteins, lipids, and waste products from the tissues. This fluid is then transported to the lymph nodes, where waste products are filtered out, and infection-fighting cells called lymphocytes are contained. Subsequently, the excess fluid in the lymph vessels is eventually returned to the bloodstream. However, when the lymph vessels are obstructed or unable to efficiently transport lymph fluid away from the tissues, localized swelling, known as lymphedema, ensues.

Lymphedema predominantly affects a single arm or leg, although in rare instances, both limbs may be involved. There are two main types of lymphedema:

1. Primary lymphedema arises from anatomical abnormalities of the lymphatic vessels and is considered a rare, hereditary condition.

2. Secondary lymphedema develops due to identifiable damage to or obstruction of normally functioning lymphatic vessels and nodes.

Globally, lymphedema is most commonly associated with filariasis, a parasitic infection. However, in the United States, lymphedema primarily occurs in women who have undergone breast cancer surgery, particularly when followed by radiation therapy. This secondary lymphedema can significantly impact an individual's quality of life and requires careful management and treatment to alleviate symptoms and prevent complications.

What leads to the development of lymphedema?

Lymphedema can develop due to various factors that disrupt the normal functioning of the lymphatic system, leading to the accumulation of lymph fluid and subsequent swelling. Some common causes and risk factors include:

1. Surgery: Surgical procedures that involve the removal or alteration of lymph nodes or lymphatic vessels can disrupt the normal flow of lymph fluid, leading to lymphedema. For example, lymphedema often occurs as a complication of cancer surgeries, such as mastectomy (removal of the breast) or lymph node dissection, particularly in cases of breast cancer, gynecological cancers, or melanoma.

2. Radiation Therapy: Radiation treatment for cancer can damage lymph nodes and lymphatic vessels, impairing their ability to transport lymph fluid effectively. This damage can occur either during or after radiation therapy and may contribute to the development of lymphedema, especially when combined with surgery.

3. Trauma or Injury: Physical trauma, such as severe burns, cuts, or other injuries, can disrupt the lymphatic system, leading to inflammation and impaired lymphatic drainage. This disruption can result in the development of secondary lymphedema in the affected area.

4. Infection: Certain infections, such as filariasis (a parasitic infection transmitted by mosquitoes), can

directly damage lymphatic vessels and nodes, leading to lymphedema. Other infections, including cellulitis or recurrent skin infections, can also contribute to the development of lymphedema by causing inflammation and scarring of the lymphatic tissues.

5. Cancer: In addition to surgery and radiation therapy, cancer itself can obstruct lymphatic vessels or invade lymph nodes, leading to lymphedema. This can occur in various types of cancer, including lymphoma, sarcoma, and metastatic cancers that spread to the lymph nodes.

6. Congenital Factors: Some individuals may be born with structural abnormalities or genetic mutations affecting the lymphatic system,

predisposing them to primary lymphedema, which can manifest at birth or later in life.

7. Obesity: Excess body weight can exert pressure on the lymphatic system, impeding lymphatic flow and increasing the risk of developing lymphedema, particularly in the lower extremities.

Overall, lymphedema is a complex condition with multiple potential causes, and its development often involves a combination of factors. Understanding these risk factors is crucial for prevention, early detection, and effective management of lymphedema.

Reasons behind Primary Lymphedema

Primary lymphedema is a condition characterized by abnormalities in an individual's lymphatic system, typically present from birth, although symptoms may not manifest until later in life. Depending on the age at which symptoms arise, three forms of primary lymphedema have been identified. The majority of primary lymphedema cases occur without any known family history of the condition.

Congenital lymphedema is evident at birth, more prevalent in females, and accounts for approximately 10-25% of all cases of primary lymphedema. Within this subgroup, some individuals exhibit a genetic inheritance pattern known as Milroy disease.

Lymphedema praecox represents the most common form of primary lymphedema. It manifests as lymphedema that becomes apparent after birth and before the age of 35, with symptoms often developing during puberty. Lymphedema praecox is four times more prevalent in females than in males.

Primary lymphedema that becomes evident after the age of 35 is termed Meige disease or lymphedema tarda, although it is less common than congenital lymphedema and lymphedema praecox.

Primary lymphedema is a rare inherited condition caused by developmental issues in the body's lymphatic vessels. Specific causes of primary lymphedema include:

- Milroy's disease (congenital lymphedema): This disorder begins in infancy and results in the abnormal formation of lymph nodes.

- Meige's disease (lymphedema praecox): This disorder often leads to lymphedema around puberty or during pregnancy, although it can occur later, up to age 35.

- Late-onset lymphedema (lymphedema tarda): This condition occurs rarely and typically starts after the age of 35.

Secondary lymphedema causes

The onset of secondary lymphedema arises when the lymphatic system, which typically functions seamlessly, encounters obstruction or damage. In the United States, breast cancer surgery, particularly when coupled with radiation therapy, emerges as the predominant trigger for this condition. Consequently, individuals often experience unilateral lymphedema in the arm on the side of the surgery. However, any surgical intervention involving the removal of regional lymph nodes or lymph vessels bears the potential to induce lymphedema. Procedures such as vein stripping, mastectomy, excision of burn scars, and peripheral vascular surgery have all been associated with this condition.

Furthermore, lymphedema can stem from trauma, burns, radiation exposure, infections, or the compression or infiltration of lymph nodes by tumors. Globally, filariasis stands as the most prevalent cause of lymphedema. This parasitic infection, caused by Wuchereria bancrofti, directly infests lymph nodes. It spreads among individuals through mosquitoes and affects millions across tropical and subtropical regions in Asia, Africa, the Western Pacific, and parts of Central and South America. Parasitic infestation inflicts damage on the lymphatic system, resulting in swelling in various parts of the body, including the arms, breasts, legs, and for men, the genital area. The affected limbs or areas may swell to several times their normal size. Additionally, the swelling, coupled with compromised lymphatic function, hampers the body's ability to combat infections.

Lymphatic filariasis ranks as a primary cause of permanent disability worldwide.

Factors that increase the likelihood of developing lymphedema

Several factors may elevate your susceptibility to developing lymphedema subsequent to cancer, as a consequence of cancer treatment, or stemming from other secondary causes. These include:

1. Advanced age: Older individuals tend to have a higher likelihood of developing lymphedema due to a variety of physiological factors associated with aging.

2. Excess weight or obesity: Being overweight or obese can place additional strain on the lymphatic system, potentially impairing its function and increasing the risk of lymphedema.

3. Rheumatoid or psoriatic arthritis: Individuals with autoimmune conditions such as rheumatoid or psoriatic arthritis may experience inflammation and swelling that can exacerbate lymphatic issues.

4. Complications: Lymphedema in your arm or leg can lead to serious complications, including:

- Infections: Lymphedema can predispose individuals to various infections, such as cellulitis (a bacterial skin infection) and lymphangitis (infection of the lymph vessels). Even minor injuries to the affected limb can serve as entry points for infection.

- Lymphangiosarcoma: In rare instances, severe and untreated cases of lymphedema can culminate in lymphangiosarcoma, a rare form of soft tissue cancer. Signs of lymphangiosarcoma may manifest as blue-red or purple marks on the skin.

These factors underscore the importance of proactive management and vigilant monitoring for individuals at risk of developing lymphedema. Early detection and intervention can significantly mitigate the risk of complications and improve overall outcomes.

CHAPTER TWO

HOW DOES LYMPHEDEMA START?

Lymphedema manifests when the lymphatic system undergoes damage, impeding the smooth return of lymph fluid to the bloodstream. This condition is particularly prevalent among individuals grappling with cancer, wherein the accumulation of lymph fluid can be attributed to various factors:

1. Surgical Procedures: Cancer surgeries, especially those involving the removal of lymph nodes, can disrupt the normal flow of lymph fluid, predisposing individuals to lymphedema.

2. Radiation Therapy: While effective in targeting cancerous cells, radiation therapy can inadvertently damage nearby lymph nodes or lymphatic vessels, exacerbating the risk of lymphedema.

3. Infections: Infections within the body can inflict harm on surrounding tissues or induce scarring, further compromising the functionality of the lymphatic system and contributing to lymphedema.

4. Coexisting Health Conditions: Certain health ailments such as heart or vascular disease, arthritis, and eczema can impede lymphatic circulation, heightening susceptibility to lymphedema.

5. Genetic Factors: Genetic alterations or mutations affecting the lymphatic system can predispose

individuals to develop lymphedema, underscoring the hereditary component of this condition.

6. Trauma or Injury: Physical trauma or injury to specific regions of the body may disrupt lymphatic pathways, impeding the normal drainage of lymph fluid and precipitating lymphedema.

7. Blood Disorders: Conditions characterized by an increased production of white blood cells, such as leukemia, can disrupt lymphatic function, contributing to the onset of lymphedema.

The multifactorial nature of lymphedema underscores the importance of comprehensive management strategies tailored to address its diverse etiological factors. By understanding the complex interplay of these contributing elements, healthcare professionals can devise targeted interventions to mitigate the impact of lymphedema and enhance the quality of life for affected individuals.

What are the visual characteristics of lymphedema?

In its initial stages, mild lymphedema may manifest as subtle sensations within the affected limb, including a sensation of heaviness, tingling, tightness, warmth, or intermittent shooting pains. These symptoms may manifest prior to any noticeable swelling in the limb. Additionally, individuals may experience other early indicators of mild lymphedema, such as:

- Reduced ability to perceive or palpate veins or tendons in the extremities.

- Tightness felt in jewelry or clothing worn on the affected limb.

- Skin redness in the affected area.

- Asymmetrical appearance of the limbs.

- Sensations of tightness or decreased flexibility in the joints.

- Slight puffiness or edema in the skin.

As lymphedema progresses from its mild form to a more moderate to severe state, the swelling in the affected limb becomes more prominent. Concurrently, the aforementioned symptoms persist and may intensify in cases of moderate or severe lymphedema. This progression underscores the importance of early detection and intervention in managing lymphedema effectively.

What are the indications and manifestations of lymphedema?

Recognizing the signs and symptoms of lymphedema is crucial for prompt identification and treatment. Lymphedema manifests through various common indicators, including:

- Swelling in specific areas of the body, such as the breast, chest, shoulder, arm, or leg.

- Changes in skin texture, which may feel tight, hard, appear reddened, or feel hot.

- Sensations of new aching, tingling, numbness, or discomfort in the affected area, often accompanied by a feeling of fullness or heaviness.

- Reduced mobility or flexibility in adjacent joints, such as the hand, wrist, or shoulder.

- Difficulty fitting limbs into clothing sleeves or pants, or experiencing challenges with buttoning garments.

- Sensations of tightness in jewelry or accessories, despite no weight gain being observed.

- While lymphedema frequently manifests in the arms or legs following surgeries or treatments affecting those areas, it can also occur in other parts of the body.

Specifically, in the context of breast cancer treatment, lymphedema can impact the breast, chest, underarm, and the arm closest to the surgical site. Similarly, treatments for cancers in the abdomen or pelvis may lead to swelling in these regions, including the abdomen, genitals, or one or both legs.

Furthermore, tumor treatments in the head and neck areas may precipitate lymphedema in the face and neck. Understanding these potential manifestations of lymphedema following cancer treatments underscores the importance of vigilance and early intervention to manage this condition effectively.

Alternative Methods for Handling Lymphedema Symptoms

In addition to following a healthy diet, you can do other things to keep lymphedema symptoms to a minimum. Combining a proper lymphedema diet with other strategies for managing lymphedema can help mitigate the condition's effects. Here are seven extra ways to manage lymphedema symptoms:

- Exercise: Regular exercise promotes joint motion, which can aid circulation and boost lymph vessel activity.
- Compression therapy: By applying pressure from the outside, compression therapy can help move and filter fluid through the lymphatic system, alleviating lymphedema symptoms.

- Massage therapy: Similar to compression therapy, massage therapy can help manually push fluid through the lymphatic system and reduce swelling.

- Proper skin care: Keeping your skin clean is key for managing lymphedema. Practice good skin hygiene and keep a close watch on your arm and leg skin so you can spot any changes or breaks in the skin early. Catching these issues early can help prevent infection.

- Wear loose clothing: Avoid wearing tight articles of clothing that could constrict your leg or arm and restrict the lymphatic system.

- Elevate your limb: Whenever you can, try to elevate the affected arm or leg above the level of your heart.

- Avoid extreme temperatures: Try not to expose the affected limb to extreme cold or heat. This means you should not apply ice or a heating pad to the swollen arm or leg.

CHAPTER THREE

WHAT ARE THE METHODS USED TO DIAGNOSE LYMPHEDEMA?

A comprehensive medical evaluation, including a detailed medical history and thorough physical examination, is essential to exclude alternative causes of limb swelling, such as edema resulting from congestive heart failure, kidney dysfunction, blood clots, or other medical conditions. Frequently, a patient's medical history, including any history of surgery or conditions involving the lymph nodes, can provide vital clues pointing to the underlying cause and aiding in the diagnosis of lymphedema.

In cases where the cause of swelling remains unclear, further diagnostic tests may be warranted to assist in determining the underlying etiology of limb swelling:

- Computed tomography (CT) or magnetic resonance imaging (MRI) scans may prove valuable in delineating the architecture of lymph nodes or identifying tumors or other abnormalities within the affected area.

- Lymphoscintigraphy is a diagnostic test involving the injection of a tracer dye into lymph vessels, followed by the observation of fluid flow using imaging technologies. This procedure can effectively highlight blockages in lymph flow, aiding in the diagnosis of lymphatic system disorders.

- Doppler ultrasound scans utilize sound waves to evaluate blood flow and can help identify the presence of a blood clot in the veins (deep vein thrombosis), which may contribute to limb swelling.

These diagnostic modalities serve as valuable tools in elucidating the underlying cause of limb swelling when clinical evaluation alone is insufficient. By employing a multidisciplinary approach and utilizing advanced diagnostic techniques, healthcare providers can effectively diagnose and manage conditions such as lymphedema, thereby improving patient outcomes and quality of life.

What potential treatments exist for lymphedema?

Lymphedema presents a challenging reality for those affected, as there is currently no definitive cure for this condition. However, various treatments are available to manage symptoms, reduce swelling, and alleviate discomfort. These therapeutic interventions aim to improve the quality of life for individuals living with lymphedema.

Compression therapy stands as a cornerstone in the management of lymphedema, effectively reducing swelling and preventing complications such as scarring. Various methods of compression treatment exist, including:

- Elastic sleeves or stockings: These garments must be properly fitted and provide gradual compression from the extremity towards the trunk to facilitate lymphatic fluid drainage.

- Bandages: Wrapping techniques involve applying bandages more tightly around the affected extremity and looser towards the trunk, encouraging lymph flow towards the body's central regions.

- Pneumatic compression devices: These devices, connected to a pump, deliver sequential compression from the extremity towards the body. While beneficial for preventing long-term scarring, they may not be suitable for all individuals, such as those with congestive heart failure, deep venous thrombosis, or certain infections.

- Manual compression: Massage techniques, known as manual lymph drainage, can be beneficial for some individuals with lymphedema.

- Exercises: Light exercises that engage and stimulate muscles in the affected area may be prescribed by healthcare providers to promote lymphatic fluid movement.

In severe cases, surgical interventions may be considered to remove excess fluid and tissue, though it's important to note that no surgical procedure can fully cure lymphedema.

Prompt and effective treatment of skin and tissue infections associated with lymphedema is crucial to prevent complications such as sepsis. Patients must vigilantly monitor for signs of infection in affected areas and seek medical attention promptly when necessary.

In regions where filariasis is prevalent, the drug diethylcarbamazine is utilized to treat this parasitic infection, which can contribute to the development of lymphedema.

While lymphedema presents challenges, a multifaceted approach to treatment can significantly improve the lives of those affected by this condition, enhancing both physical comfort and overall well-being.

Is it possible to prevent lymphedema?

While primary lymphedema cannot be outright prevented, proactive measures can be taken to mitigate the risk of developing lymphedema, particularly for individuals predisposed to secondary lymphedema, such as those who have undergone cancer surgery or radiation treatment. These precautionary steps aim to reduce the likelihood of lymphedema onset:

1. Elevate the affected arm or leg above the level of the heart whenever feasible to facilitate lymphatic drainage.

2. Refrain from wearing tight or restrictive garments or jewelry, and avoid the use of blood pressure cuffs on the affected limb.

3. Avoid applying heat pads to the affected area and steer clear of hot tubs, steam baths, and similar heat sources.

4. Maintain adequate hydration levels to support overall bodily function, including lymphatic circulation.

5. Steer clear of heavy lifting and strenuous activity involving the affected limb, while still encouraging light, regular physical activity.

6. Minimize the burden on the affected arm by avoiding carrying heavy purses or bags.

7. Adhere to diligent and meticulous skin hygiene practices to prevent infection and skin irritation.

8. Take precautions to avoid insect bites and sunburn, which can exacerbate lymphatic issues and skin sensitivity.

By incorporating these proactive measures into daily routines, individuals at risk for secondary lymphedema can potentially reduce the likelihood of developing this condition and maintain better overall lymphatic health.

CHAPTER FOUR

DIET AND LYMPHEDEMA

Dietary recommendations for lymphedema management encompass a multifaceted approach aimed at optimizing nutritional intake while mitigating factors that may exacerbate symptoms. Emphasizing the consumption of predominantly whole foods forms the cornerstone of this dietary strategy, particularly focusing on a diverse array of rainbow-colored fruits and vegetables.

Whole foods take precedence in this dietary plan due to their inherent nutritional value and absence of added sugars, salts, unhealthy fats, soy, or artificial additives, which could potentially contribute to inflammation and fluid retention. Gluten-free grains, including brown rice, oats, quinoa, and wild rice, feature prominently, offering valuable sources of complex carbohydrates and fiber while catering to individuals with sensitivities or intolerances.

In the realm of dairy alternatives, almond, coconut, and hemp milk emerge as preferred options, providing essential nutrients without the added sugars often found in sweetened dairy milk products. Fermented foods, such as kefir, yogurt, pickles, and kimchi, are advocated for their probiotic content, which supports gut health and may confer benefits for individuals managing lymphedema.

By incorporating these dietary principles into daily eating habits, individuals with lymphedema can not only support their overall health and well-being but also potentially alleviate symptoms associated with this condition. Additionally, consulting with a healthcare professional or registered dietitian can provide personalized guidance tailored to individual needs and preferences, ensuring optimal dietary management of lymphedema.

Are there certain foods that ought to be restricted?

Certain food items should be consumed in moderation to maintain a balanced diet and promote overall health. These include:

- Nuts: While nuts are nutritious and rich in healthy fats, they are also calorie-dense, so it's important to consume them in limited quantities to avoid excess calorie intake.

- Dairy: Dairy products such as milk, cheese, and yogurt are excellent sources of calcium and protein. However, they can also be high in saturated fats and calories, so moderation is key.

- Eggs: Eggs are a versatile and nutrient-rich food, but they are also relatively high in cholesterol. Enjoying them in moderation can help balance their nutritional benefits with potential health risks.

- Poultry and Meat: Lean poultry and meat are valuable sources of protein, vitamins, and minerals. However, excessive consumption can contribute to high cholesterol levels and other health issues, so it's advisable to limit intake.

- Oils and Condiments: While oils and condiments add flavor to meals, they are often high in calories and may contain unhealthy fats. Using them sparingly can help manage calorie intake and promote heart health.

- Dried Fruit, Sugar, and Real Maple Syrup: These sweeteners are concentrated sources of sugar and calories. While they can add sweetness to dishes and snacks, consuming them only occasionally can help prevent excess sugar intake and maintain blood sugar levels.

- Wine: Red wine, in particular, contains antioxidants and may offer certain health benefits when consumed in moderation. However, excessive alcohol consumption can have negative effects on health, so it's best to limit wine intake to no more than three servings per week.

By enjoying these foods in moderation and incorporating a variety of nutrient-dense options into your diet, you can strike a balance between indulgence and healthy eating to support your overall well-being.

Are there particular foods that should be completely avoided?

Certain foods are best consumed sparingly or avoided altogether to maintain optimal health, particularly for individuals dealing with lymphedema. These foods include:

- Grains containing gluten: Found in a variety of products such as bread, cakes, cookies, breakfast cereals, crackers, pasta, pies, etc. It's advised to avoid gluten-free food substitutes as well, which may still contain ingredients like cornstarch, rice starch, or potato starch.

- Processed meats: Meats preserved with salt, nitrates, or nitrites, as well as meat substitutes containing gluten or highly processed soy, should be limited or avoided.

- Beverages: It's recommended to steer clear of sweetened drinks (both sugar and artificially sweetened), soft drinks, teas, coffee-based beverages, fruit drinks, soy milk, beer, liquor, mixed drinks, and wine coolers.

Maintaining a healthy weight is crucial for individuals with lymphedema, as excess body mass can exacerbate symptoms. The risk of lymphedema increases with a high body mass index (BMI) due to the added strain on the lymphatic system. Increased adipose tissue makes it more challenging for the body to manage lymphatic fluid, leading to further inflammation.

There are numerous misconceptions regarding dietary recommendations for lymphedema management. Some suggest avoiding sodium, while others advocate for reducing protein or fluid intake. With conflicting advice, it can be challenging to discern the best approach.

First and foremost, there's no one-size-fits-all meal plan to alleviate lymphedema symptoms. However, adopting certain eating habits can promote overall health, control swelling, and help the body manage the stresses associated with lymphedema.

Let's delve into some dietary considerations:

Sodium:

While there's no definitive evidence supporting a low-sodium diet's efficacy in controlling lymphedema, limiting salt intake has proven beneficial for some individuals. Sodium plays a crucial role in regulating various bodily functions, including blood pressure and fluid balance. However, excessive salt consumption can lead to fluid retention and hypertension.

What you can do:

- Aim to consume no more than 1,500-2,300 milligrams of salt per day.

- Incorporate fresh fruits and vegetables, which naturally contain appropriate sodium levels.

Protein:

Lymphedema involves the accumulation of high-protein fluid in tissue spaces, but this doesn't correlate with the protein content of your diet. Proteins are essential for tissue repair and muscle maintenance. They serve as building blocks for the body and play a vital role in hormone and antibody production.

What you can do:

- Obtain protein from a variety of sources, not just meat, and limit dietary fat intake.

- Opt for easily digestible proteins such as chicken, fish, and tofu.

Hydration:

Maintaining adequate fluid levels in the body helps eliminate toxins from the blood. Contrary to popular belief, reducing fluid intake to alleviate lymphedema swelling is ineffective. In fact, the protein-rich lymph attracts more fluid from other body parts, exacerbating swelling in the affected area.

What you can do:

- Drink eight 8-ounce glasses of water daily, increasing fluid intake in hot weather or dry conditions.

- Avoid caffeine and alcohol, which act as mild diuretics and reduce body fluid levels.

Body Weight:

Excess weight places additional strain on the lymphatic system and increases fluid accumulation in already swollen tissues. As fat cells enlarge and multiply with weight gain, the lymphatic flow becomes more restricted, leading to stagnation and further swelling. Additionally, obesity is associated with various health issues like diabetes, high blood pressure, and heart problems.

What you can do:

- Maintain a healthy, ideal body weight.

- Limit or avoid fatty foods and those high in cholesterol.

- Increase consumption of low-sodium or high-fiber foods.

- Replace processed foods with fresh and raw potassium-rich options like fruits and vegetables.

- Follow a balanced, healthy diet comprising whole grains, fruits, vegetables, and fish, which supports the body's immune system and aids in infection prevention and treatment.

- Consider taking vitamins and/or supplements, especially a multivitamin, vitamin C for collagen formation, vitamin A for increased cell development, and zinc for wound healing (consult with your doctor before starting any new supplements or vitamins).

By adopting these dietary guidelines, individuals with lymphedema can take proactive steps towards managing their condition and improving overall health.

What stages does lymphedema progress through?

The severity of lymphedema, a condition characterized by swelling due to a compromised lymphatic system, is often delineated by its stages, each indicating varying degrees of progression and symptomatology:

• Stage 0: Absence of visible swelling, yet subtle symptoms such as a sensation of heaviness or fullness in the affected area, or tightness of the skin may be experienced.

• Stage 1: Manifestation of swelling in the affected area, with noticeable increases in size or stiffness of the limb or region. Swelling typically diminishes when the affected limb is elevated.

• Stage 2: Presence of more pronounced swelling compared to Stage 1, which does not subside upon elevation of the limb. The affected area may feel hard and exhibit a larger size than in Stage 1.

• Stage 3: Severe swelling exceeding that of Stage 2, to the extent that lifting or moving the limb without assistance becomes challenging. The skin may become dry and thickened, and fluid leakage or blister formation may occur.

With progression to later stages, particularly Stage 2 or 3, there is an increased risk of infection in the affected area, necessitating prompt medical attention.

Early stages (Stages 0 and 1) of lymphedema are often reversible with appropriate management, while later stages (Stages 2 and 3) may exhibit reduced responsiveness to treatment interventions. Thus, timely consultation with a healthcare provider upon noticing any concerning symptoms is imperative.

Additionally, the onset of cellulitis, an infection in the tissues beneath the skin, poses a significant concern in individuals with lymphedema. Cellulitis can exacerbate lymphedema and requires immediate medical attention. Signs and symptoms of cellulitis include redness, warmth, pain, and possibly cracking or peeling of the skin in the affected area, accompanied by fever and flu-like symptoms. Repeated occurrences may necessitate antibiotic therapy to manage the condition effectively.

Given the interplay between lymphedema and cellulitis, vigilant monitoring for signs and symptoms is crucial in individuals with lymphedema to promptly identify and address any potential complications.

CHAPTER FIVE

WHAT CONSTITUTES THE LYMPHATIC SYSTEM?

The lymphatic system, an integral component of the body's immune defense, comprises a complex network of lymph nodes, vessels, and organs collaborating harmoniously to gather and transport clear lymph fluid throughout the body's tissues, eventually returning it to the bloodstream. This intricate system bears resemblance to the venous system, which collects blood from remote areas of the body, such as the hands and arms, and transports it back to the heart.

Lymph fluid, coursing through the body, carries proteins, salts, water, and crucially, white blood cells, which play a pivotal role in combating infections and maintaining immune function.

Lymph vessels, equipped with one-way valves, cooperate with the body's musculature to facilitate the movement of fluid through the body while regulating its flow. These vessels ensure efficient circulation of lymph fluid, aiding in waste removal and immune surveillance.

Scattered along the lymphatic vessels are small, bean-sized structures known as lymph nodes. These glands function as filtration hubs, intercepting foreign substances, such as tumor cells and infectious agents, and orchestrating immune responses. Distributed throughout various regions of the body, including the neck, armpit, chest, abdomen (belly), and groin, lymph nodes act as sentinel stations safeguarding against invaders.

Moreover, the lymphatic system encompasses additional organs vital to immune function, such as the tonsils, adenoids, spleen, and thymus. Together, these components form an intricate network that plays a fundamental role in preserving health and defending the body against disease.

What is Lipedema?

Lipedema, alternatively spelled as lipoedema, represents a condition distinct from lymphedema, characterized by the abnormal accumulation of inflamed fat cells, predominantly affecting women. Its hallmark features include discomfort and irregular sensations within the tissues of the lower limbs, hips, and buttocks, with occasional involvement of the arms, albeit less frequently observed.

Individuals afflicted with lipedema typically exhibit disproportionately enlarged hips and legs relative to their waist and upper body regions. Although the lower extremities may appear swollen, their feet generally maintain a normal size. The application of pressure on these enlarged limbs often induces considerable pain, rendering procedures such as leg massages and the wearing of compression stockings uncomfortable for lipedema patients. Moreover, hormonal fluctuations, such as those occurring during menstrual cycles, have been reported to exacerbate symptoms.

Furthermore, it is not uncommon for individuals with lipedema to concurrently experience venous diseases, further complicating their condition and therapeutic approach. Nonetheless, with appropriate management strategies, including tailored treatment plans, symptoms associated with lipedema can be effectively mitigated, enhancing the overall quality of life for affected individuals.

What are the characteristics of "typical" lipedema? What symptoms typically manifest with this condition?

The classic presentation of lipedema is often described as a woman with a small upper body and disproportionately fatty lower body. However, delving into this condition reveals a myriad of nuances and variations beyond this stereotypical image. Lipedema, a condition primarily affecting women, but occasionally observed in men with hormonal imbalances or liver disease, manifests in diverse ways, with symptoms that evolve over the progression of the disease and can overlap with those of other conditions.

Let's begin by examining the classic symptoms:

Classic symptoms of lipedema:

Lipedema predominantly affects the lower body, typically presenting as excessive fat accumulation in the lower limbs while the upper body remains relatively thin. If there's proportional obesity in the upper body, lipedema is unlikely. However, about 30% of patients may also experience involvement of the arms, primarily affecting the upper arms.

Unlike typical weight gain, the ankles and feet remain unaffected in lipedema. Instead of fat accumulation, a characteristic collar of fat can often be observed just above the ankles.

Lipedema exhibits symmetrical fat accumulation, affecting both sides of the body similarly. The pattern of fat distribution can vary widely, leading to leg shapes resembling columnar trunks or presenting as lumpy. Fat deposits may also occur below the knee.

Fat areas in lipedema feel abnormal and are painful to the touch. Unlike normal fat, lipedema fat areas tend to be tender upon pressure and are susceptible to bruising. Moreover, these fat deposits can cause discomfort even without external pressure, and the skin may lose its elasticity.

However, the symptoms of lipedema can be more intricate:

Lipedema can affect men in rare instances. Moreover, it is not a static condition but rather progressive, meaning symptoms typically start mildly and worsen over time if preventative measures aren't taken.

Early stages of lipedema can be challenging to differentiate from simple weight gain in otherwise healthy individuals. However, advanced stages may manifest additional characteristics, including symptoms akin to the chronic swelling condition known as lymphedema. Thus, the ease of correctly diagnosing lipedema changes with the stage of presentation.

Understanding the origins and progression of lipedema is essential for accurate diagnosis and effective management of this condition, as its diverse presentations and evolving symptoms demand a nuanced approach to care.

Characteristics that distinguish lipedema from lymphedema include:

1. Pain is a predominant complaint among individuals with lipedema, often exacerbated by touch, particularly on the legs. Simple actions like a cat walking on their legs can evoke discomfort and sensitivity.

2. Bruising and subcutaneous bleeding are common occurrences in lipedema patients, resulting from impacts or even spontaneous events. The fragility of blood vessels within affected tissues can contribute to these manifestations.

3. Unlike lymphedema, infections are less common in areas affected solely by lipedema. However, once lymphedema swelling develops, the risk of infections increases, highlighting a distinct characteristic between the two conditions.

4. In the early stages of lipedema, there's a striking contrast between the upper body, which may remain slim, and the accumulation of fat from the hips down to the ankles. Remarkably, the feet remain unaffected, with swelling ceasing at the ankles, a phenomenon evident in negative skin-fold tests (Stemmer sign) on the feet or toes.

5. Weight gain in lipedema typically occurs symmetrically on both legs, from the hips to the ankles. This symmetry distinguishes it from swelling resulting from lymphedema.

6. Weight loss in lipedema is restricted to areas unaffected by the condition. Therefore, if lipedema coexists with obesity, weight loss may be noticeable in regions other than the legs.

7. Leg swelling in lipedema tends to worsen during prolonged standing, periods of heightened temperatures, and in the latter part of the day. While some individuals experience reduced swelling during sleep, others do not benefit from this phenomenon.

8. Initially, lipedema skin appears smooth, but over time, the development of fatty lumps or nodules within affected tissues leads to a lumpy appearance.

9. In advanced stages of lipedema, larger rounded fat deposits called lobules develop, resulting in irregularly shaped legs that can impact posture and walking mechanics. This transformation alters the contours of the legs, contributing to functional limitations and aesthetic concerns.

Phases of Lipedema

Lipedema progresses through distinct stages, each characterized by unique changes in the appearance and distribution of fat tissue:

1. Stage 1: In this initial stage, individuals typically exhibit a normal skin surface with localized areas of enlarged fat deposits.

2. Stage 2: As lipedema advances, the skin becomes uneven, often displaying indentations known as cellulite. The surface of the skin takes on a lumpy appearance resembling a mattress, with fat globules protruding between thickened connective fibers known as fibrotic septa.

3. Stage 3: At this stage, large protrusions of tissue may develop, causing noticeable deformations, particularly in areas such as the thighs and around the knees.

4. Stage 4: Lipedema may progress to a more severe stage, often accompanied by lymphedema, termed lipo-lymphedema. This stage is characterized by abnormal fat accumulation not only in the lower extremities but also in the hands, feet, trunk, and head.

As lipedema advances through these stages, individuals may experience varying degrees of discomfort, mobility limitations, and psychological distress. Early recognition and intervention are essential for managing symptoms and improving quality of life for those affected by this condition.

CHAPTER SIX

DIFFERENT CATEGORIES OF LIPEDEMA

The classification of lipedema is primarily determined by the distribution pattern of excess fat in the body. There are five recognized types:

1. Type I: Predominantly affects the buttocks and hips, often referred to as the "saddlebag" or "jodhpur" phenomenon due to the characteristic accumulation of fat in these areas.

2. Type II: Extends from the buttocks down to the knees, with the development of folds of fat around the inner side of the knees contributing to the characteristic appearance.

3. Type III: Involves fat accumulation extending from the buttocks down to the ankles, leading to a significant increase in lower limb size and shape.

4. Type IV: Targets the arms, resulting in disproportionate fat deposition in this region, which may lead to discomfort and functional impairment.

5. Type V: Primarily affects the legs, resulting in pronounced enlargement and distortion of the

lower limbs, often accompanied by discomfort and mobility issues.

These distinct patterns of fat distribution characterize the various types of lipedema, providing valuable diagnostic information for healthcare professionals and guiding treatment strategies tailored to address the specific needs of individuals with this condition.

What leads to the progression of lipedema?

Here is a detailed explanation of how adipose tissue functions and how lipedema might disrupt normal physiological processes, leading to a progressively worsening condition. While a comprehensive understanding of lipedema remains elusive, a general framework has emerged to elucidate the causes and progression of this condition. As you delve into the intricacies of lipedema, you will find that excess fluid accumulation plays a pivotal role.

Adipose tissue consists of cells known as adipocytes, which are heavily reliant on adequate blood flow. These cells synthesize, store, and metabolize fat. Unlike other cells, fat cells do not multiply significantly in number during weight gain; rather, they increase in size. They play a crucial role in maintaining the balance of fats and carbohydrates in the bloodstream, supported by a dense network of blood capillaries that supply them with nutrients and oxygen. Consequently, there is a substantial exchange of fluid within fat tissue.

Fat tissue is under constant pressure to regulate fluid balance; otherwise, swelling occurs. A considerable amount of fluid continuously enters fat tissue and must be removed through the venous and lymphatic systems. These systems work collaboratively to drain accumulating fluid. However, if these drainage systems are inadequate, swelling ensues. For instance, chronic swelling conditions like lymphedema result from lymphatic damage or abnormalities.

In patients with lipedema, fluid circulation appears to be abnormal, potentially exacerbating swelling. Observations indicate that the blood vessels supplying fat deposits in individuals with lipedema are fragile and leaky, as are the small lymphatic vessels. This suggests that fat tissue in lipedema patients may be prone to fluid accumulation. Additionally, there seems to be reduced skin elasticity in individuals with lipedema, further increasing susceptibility to fluid retention.

Gravity exacerbates fluid accumulation in the lower body, particularly in fat tissue. This increases the demands on the venous and lymphatic systems responsible for draining fluid from this region. Consequently, individuals with lipedema are more likely to accumulate excess fluid in their legs, leading to leg swelling.

Chronic swelling appears to promote fat accumulation, creating a potential feedback loop. Inflammation associated with swelling has been shown to promote fat accumulation and damage to fat tissue. This phenomenon has been observed in patients with late-stage lymphedema, suggesting a similar mechanism in lipedema.

As tissue expands, particularly fat tissue, it attracts more blood flow. However, the lymphatic drainage system has a finite capacity to remove fluid from tissues. Chronic obesity alone can overwhelm the lymphatic system, leading to secondary lymphedema. Excessive fat accumulation caused by lipedema can exacerbate fluid accumulation in the lower body, potentially exceeding the capacity of the local lymphatic system and resulting in swelling.

This comprehensive view of lipedema underscores the complex interplay between fluid dynamics, fat metabolism, and tissue integrity. It suggests that an inability to maintain fluid balance within fat tissue may be a central driver of lipedema, leading to the characteristic swelling and fat deposition observed in affected individuals.

Manifestations and Phases of Lipedema Lipolymphedema

As the progression of lipedema unfolds, the symptomatic landscape undergoes notable shifts. In its advanced stages, the condition manifests as an accumulation of excess fat alongside progressive insufficiency and damage to the lymphatic system. This cascade of events precipitates the emergence of secondary lymphedema, characterized by fluid retention within the affected area. This combined condition, termed "lipo-lymphedema," presents a fusion of symptoms from both lipedema and lower-limb lymphedema, including swelling below the ankles and in the feet, which are not typically observed in isolated lipedema cases.

Conversely, individuals with advanced, untreated cases of lymphedema may experience tissue hardening due to fibrosis, loss of skin elasticity, and additional fat deposition. Consequently, advanced presentations of both lipedema and lymphedema may exhibit overlapping symptoms. Adding to the diagnostic complexity, prolonged obesity in otherwise healthy individuals also appears to trigger the development of secondary lymphedema, along with its associated symptoms.

Given these intricacies, distinguishing between lipedema, advanced lipedema (lipo-lymphedema), advanced lymphedema, obesity-induced secondary lymphedema, or mere obesity requires a thorough understanding of a patient's symptom history and how these symptoms have evolved over time. In essence, an accurate diagnosis of lipedema necessitates a comprehensive grasp of a patient's symptom trajectory within the context of the three stages of the disease progression.

Indications and manifestations of the three phases of lipoedema:

Stage I Lipedema marks the initial phase of this condition, characterized by subtle yet crucial indicators that may not be immediately discernible solely by appearance. While outward signs alone may not definitively distinguish between lipedema and normal adiposity, a comprehensive assessment encompassing various characteristics of Stage I lipedema can effectively assist in the identification or exclusion of the condition in many instances.

Distinctive Features of Stage I Lipedema:

- Legs exhibit an excess accumulation of fat disproportionate to the upper body, with weight loss efforts typically failing to reduce fat in the affected area. This adiposity affects both legs uniformly and is evenly distributed from the hips down to the ankles. Fat pads may manifest above and below the knees, obscuring the natural contours of the legs.

- Absence of excess fat or swelling in the ankles or feet.

- Skin maintains a healthy appearance and remains unblemished.

- Fat deposits elicit pain upon pressure application. Unlike healthy individuals with thicker legs or those with lymphedema, patients with lipedema often experience discomfort when pressure is exerted on fat deposits. Some individuals may even report spontaneous pain without external stimuli, which often does not respond to over-the-counter pain medication.

- Abnormality of the fat tissue. Fat deposits associated with lipedema exhibit aberrations beyond mere excess, such as heightened susceptibility to bruising due to microvascular fragility, inflammatory processes exacerbating complications, and susceptibility to bacterial skin infections like cellulitis. Although soft to the touch, the fat may feel distinct from fat in other body areas and may contain small, evenly dispersed fat nodules.

- Absence of Stemmer's sign. Stemmer's sign, negative in Stage I lipedema, allows for the pinching and lifting of skin on the toes without resistance. This test seeks to detect swelling and fibrotic tissue in the feet, which do not typically occur in Stage I Lipedema. Stemmer's sign is positive in cases of lymphedema affecting the feet.

- Lack of pitting upon pressure application to the fat area. This test, another indicator for swelling, involves pressing the area with a finger or thumb. If an indentation remains, gradually filling in and disappearing, it suggests fluid-based swelling rather than fat deposition.

- Occasional temporary swelling in the ankles or feet at day's end, resolving with elevation or rest, is possible in Stage I lipedema.

By recognizing and understanding these nuanced characteristics, healthcare providers can better identify and manage Stage I Lipedema, facilitating timely interventions and personalized care strategies to address patients' needs effectively.

CHAPTER SEVEN

HOW IS LIPEDEMA DIAGNOSED?

Lipedema, characterized by the abnormal accumulation of fat in the hips and legs, is primarily diagnosed through clinical observation rather than specific testing procedures. Identifying signs of lipedema often involves recognizing distinctive patterns of fat distribution and associated symptoms. Individuals with lipedema may exhibit a predisposition to store fat in the lower body, resulting in disproportionate enlargement of the hips and legs compared to the upper body.

One hallmark of lipedema is the tendency for fat to accumulate unevenly, forming irregular clusters or "clumps" in areas such as the outer hips and thighs. This localized fat deposition can lead to a visibly asymmetrical lower body shape, contributing to physical discomfort and emotional distress.

Moreover, weight loss efforts typically affect the upper body first, exacerbating the perceived disproportionality between the upper and lower body regions. Despite attempts to reduce overall body weight, individuals with lipedema often find that their legs remain disproportionately large, highlighting the unique challenges associated with this condition.

In addition to alterations in fat distribution, individuals with lipedema commonly experience various physical symptoms. The legs may feel tender to the touch, and even light pressure can elicit significant discomfort or pain. Patients may also describe peculiar sensations in the legs, such as a "creepy-crawly" feeling, further complicating their experience of the condition.

Furthermore, restless legs syndrome, characterized by an uncontrollable urge to move the legs, may disrupt sleep and exacerbate discomfort in individuals with lipedema. This nocturnal restlessness adds another layer of complexity to the management of symptoms and overall quality of life.

Interestingly, conventional treatments like diuretics, often prescribed to reduce swelling, typically yield minimal improvement in leg size or perceived swelling for individuals with lipedema. This underscores the distinct pathophysiology of lipedema compared to other conditions involving fluid retention.

Moreover, familial clustering of lipedema suggests a genetic predisposition, with affected individuals often sharing similar body shapes characterized by disproportionately large lower bodies. Understanding these familial patterns can aid in both diagnosis and the identification of potential genetic factors contributing to the development of lipedema.

In summary, lipedema presents a multifaceted challenge characterized by distinctive fat distribution patterns, associated symptoms, and familial tendencies. Recognition of these features is crucial for accurate diagnosis and the development of targeted management strategies aimed at alleviating symptoms and improving quality of life for individuals affected by this condition.

With the array of symptoms present, what are the typical methods used to diagnose lipoedema?

In general, lipedema is a condition that is not widely recognized, both in terms of its prevalence and its diagnostic accuracy. While it's been reported that approximately 11% of women may suffer from this condition, our appreciation and understanding of it remain quite limited. In fact, pinning down the exact prevalence is challenging; published estimates vary significantly, ranging from 1 in 72,000 to 1 in 5 women.

The lack of widespread awareness about lipedema often leads to misdiagnoses, with the condition commonly mistaken for simple obesity or primary lymphedema, a congenital form of lymphedema affecting both sides of the body. Compounding this issue is the absence of standardized protocols or diagnostic tests specifically designed for identifying lipedema at present.

Diagnosing lipedema and its variant, lipo-lymphedema, relies heavily on physical examination through palpation, coupled with a thorough review of the patient's clinical and family history. Family history can offer valuable insights since lipedema has a hereditary component, with an estimated 15% of individuals with lipedema having a family member affected by the condition.

Thus, rather than relying solely on diagnostic tests, a comprehensive assessment encompassing physical examination and familial context proves most effective in identifying and understanding lipedema. This multifaceted approach is crucial for accurate diagnosis and appropriate management, given the complexities and nuances associated with this often underrecognized condition.

Treatment for lipedema

The initial step toward effectively managing lipedema involves obtaining an accurate diagnosis. Unfortunately, many healthcare providers lack familiarity with this condition, which can result in misdiagnosis or delayed diagnosis for affected individuals. If you suspect that you may have lipedema but have not received a formal diagnosis, seeking consultation with a vascular specialist is advisable. These medical professionals possess specialized knowledge regarding various causes of leg pain and are equipped to conduct thorough evaluations to either confirm or rule out lipedema as the underlying cause of your symptoms.

Typically, treatment for lipedema incorporates several strategies aimed at alleviating symptoms and promoting overall well-being:

1. Compression Therapy: One of the primary interventions for managing lipedema involves the use of compression garments. These garments exert pressure on the affected limbs, facilitating the movement of inflammatory substances out of the tissues and preventing their re-accumulation. While the consistent use of well-fitting compression garments can help reduce the enlargement and remodeling of affected limbs, finding the most suitable option may require some

trial and error due to potential discomfort. Options range from knee-high socks to thigh-high stockings and leggings, with some individuals finding leggings particularly comfortable due to their lack of tight bands around the legs. Additionally, pneumatic compression pumps, which gently massage the legs by inflating sleeves with air, can aid in lymphatic fluid flow and provide relief for some patients.

2. Dietary Modifications: Adopting an anti-inflammatory diet can benefit individuals with lipedema by reducing inflammation and promoting overall health. This entails avoiding processed and pre-made foods in favor of whole-food, homemade alternatives. Opting for a plant-based diet rich in fruits, vegetables, and lean proteins while minimizing saturated fats and meats can help manage symptoms. Incorporating natural anti-

inflammatory ingredients such as garlic and turmeric into cooking or supplementation may further enhance the effectiveness of dietary interventions. Weight management is also crucial in slowing disease progression, as excess fat can exacerbate symptoms. It's important to note, however, that while weight loss can be beneficial, it does not cure the discomfort associated with lipedema and should not be considered as a standalone therapy.

3. Exercise: Engaging in regular, low-impact exercise can assist in manually moving inflammatory products out of the tissues and may help alleviate symptoms associated with hormonal fluctuations.

4. Liposuction: For some patients, traditional weight loss methods may prove insufficient in alleviating pain and reducing limb size. In such cases, liposuction presents a viable option for achieving better outcomes. By removing the inflamed fat cells, liposuction has shown significant effectiveness in many patients. However, it's essential to note that insurance coverage for this procedure is often limited, and it should only be considered after consulting with a plastic surgeon experienced in treating lipedema.

5. Vascular Care: In addition to addressing lipedema-specific concerns, it's important to evaluate and manage any associated vascular conditions that may contribute to symptoms. Some patients with lipedema may also experience deep or superficial vein disease, which can exacerbate discomfort and swelling. Signs of vein disease

include spider or varicose veins, leg swelling, discoloration, heaviness or fatigue of the legs, itching, or restlessness. Treating vein disease can help alleviate some leg symptoms and improve overall quality of life.

By employing a comprehensive approach that encompasses various treatment modalities, individuals with lipedema can effectively manage their condition and improve their overall well-being. However, it's crucial to consult with healthcare professionals specializing in lipedema to develop a personalized treatment plan tailored to individual needs and circumstances.

CHAPTER EIGHT

RECIPES FOR COMBATING LYMPHEDEMA AND LIPEDEMA.

Super-greens frittata:

Ingredients

1 cup fresh basil leaves

1/2 cup fresh flat-leaf parsley leaves

3 green onions, roughly chopped

2 zucchini, roughly chopped

80g baby spinach, plus extra to serve

2 tbsp extra virgin olive oil

8 eggs

1/2 cup plain Greek-style yoghurt

250g mixed mushrooms, sliced (see notes)

200g broccoli, cut into florets

2 garlic cloves, thinly sliced

1/4 cup pepitas and sunflower seed mix (see notes)

1 tbsp lemon zest

2 tsp fresh tarragon leaves, finely chopped

Parmesan, or vegetarian hard cheese, finely grated, to serve

Directions

Step 1: Place basil, parsley, green onion, zucchini and spinach in a food processor. Process until finely chopped.

Step 2: Heat 1/2 the oil in a 22cm (base) ovenproof frying pan over medium-high heat. Add zucchini mixture. Cook, stirring occasionally, for 5 minutes or until tender and any liquid has evaporated.

Step 3: Whisk eggs and yoghurt. Season with salt and pepper. Add to zucchini mixture in pan. Stir until well combined. Reduce heat to low. Cook for 8 to 10 minutes or until almost set (mixture will wobble slightly in the centre).

Step 4: Meanwhile, heat remaining oil in a wok or frying pan over high heat. Add mushroom and broccoli. Cook, tossing, for 6 minutes or until beginning to char. Add garlic, seed mix, lemon zest and tarragon. Cook, tossing, for 2 minutes or until seeds are toasted. Remove from heat.

Step 5: Preheat grill on high. Grill frittata for 3 minutes or until top is golden and frittata is set. Top with broccoli mixture, extra baby spinach and parmesan. Serve.

Baked Lemon Garlic Salmon Recipe

Ingredients

For Salmon:

2 lb salmon fillet

Kosher salt

Extra virgin olive oil (I used Early Harvest Greek extra virgin olive oil)

½ lemon, sliced into rounds

Parsley for garnish

For Lemon-Garlic Sauce:

Zest of 1 large lemon

Juice of 2 lemons

3 tbsp extra virgin olive oil (I used Early Harvest Greek extra virgin olive oil)

5 garlic cloves, chopped

2 tsp dry oregano

1 tsp sweet paprika

½ tsp black pepper

Directions

Heat oven to 375 degrees F.

Make the lemon-garlic sauce. In a small bowl or measuring cup, mix together the lemon juice, lemon zest, extra virgin olive oil, garlic, oregano, paprika and black pepper. Give the sauce a good whisk.

Prepare a sheet pan lined with a large piece of foil (should be large enough to fold over salmon). Brush top of the foil with extra virgin olive oil.

Now, pat salmon dry and season well on both sides with kosher salt. Place it on the foiled sheetpan. Top with lemon garlic sauce (make sure to spread the sauce evenly.)

Fold foil over the salmon (seam-side up). Bake for 15 to 20 minutes until salmon is almost completely cooked through at the thickest part (cooking time will vary based on the thickness of your fish. If your salmon is thinner, check several minutes early to ensure your salmon does not overcook. If your piece is very thick, 1 ½ or more inches, it may take a bit longer.)

Carefully remove from oven and open foil to uncover the top of the salmon. Place under the broiler briefly, about 3 minutes or so. Watch closely as it broils to make sure it doesn't overcook and the garlic does not burn.)

Notes

Cook's Tip: Once you remove salmon from the oven, if it still appears underdone, you can wrap the foil back over the top and let it rest for a few minutes. Don't leave it too long, Salmon can easily go from under-cooked to way over-cooked quickly.

How do you know if Salmon is ready? When the salmon flakes easily with a fork, it's ready. If you like, you can use an instant read thermometer to check the fish for doneness. The USDA recommends a minimum internal temperature of 145°F, which should be measured at the thickest part of the fillet

Easy Greek-Style Eggplant Recipe:

This simple vegan eggplant recipe with chickpeas and tomatoes is all the comfort! And you'll love the Greek flavors thanks to a little extra virgin olive oil and a combination of warm spices including oregano, paprika, and a pinch of cinnamon.

Ingredients

1.5 lb eggplant, cut into cubes

Kosher salt

Extra Virgin Olive Oil (I used Private Reserve Greek EVOO)

1 large yellow onion, chopped

1 green bell pepper, stem and innards removed, diced

1 carrot, chopped

6 large garlic cloves, minced

2 dry bay leaves

1 to 1 ½ tsp sweet paprika OR smoked paprika

1 tsp organic ground coriander

1 tsp dry oregano

¾ tsp ground cinnamon

½ tsp organic ground turmeric

½ tsp black pepper

1 28-oz can chopped tomato

2 15-oz cans chickpeas, reserve the canning liquid

Fresh herbs such as parsley and mint for garnish

Directions

Heat oven to 400 degrees F.

Place eggplant cubes in a colander over a large bowl or directly over your sink, and sprinkle with salt. Set aside for 20 minutes or so to allow eggplant to "sweat out" any bitterness. Rinse with water and pat dry.

In a large braiser, heat ¼ cup extra virgin olive oil over medium-high until shimmering but not smoking. Add onions, peppers, and chopped carrot. Cook for 2-3 minutes, stirring regularly, then add garlic, bay leaf, spices, and a dash of salt. Cook another minute, stirring until fragrant.

Now add eggplant, chopped tomato, chickpeas, and reserved chickpea liquid. Stir to combine.

Bring to a rolling boil for 10 minutes or so. Stir often. Remove from stove top, cover and transfer to oven.

Cook in oven for 45 minutes until eggplant is fully cooked through to very tender. (While eggplant is braising, be sure to check once or twice to see if more liquid is needed. If so, remove from oven briefly and stir in about ½ cup of water at a time.)

When eggplant is ready, remove from oven and add a generous drizzle of Private Reserve EVOO, garnish with fresh herbs (parsley or mint). Serve hot or at room temperature with a side of Greek yogurt or even Tzatziki sauce and pita bread.

Shakshuka

Egg shakshuka is a simple one-skillet dish of gently poached eggs in a tasty mixture of simmering tomatoes, green peppers, onions and garlic. A few spices are added, and they may vary slightly from one recipe to another.

Ingredients

Extra virgin olive oil (I used Private Reserve EVOO)

1 large yellow onion, chopped

2 green peppers, chopped

2 garlic cloves, peeled, chopped

1 tsp ground coriander

1 tsp sweet paprika

½ tsp ground cumin

Pinch red pepper flakes (optional)

Salt and pepper

6 Vine-ripe tomatoes, chopped (about 6 cups chopped tomatoes)

½ cup tomato sauce

6 large eggs

¼ cup chopped fresh parsley leaves (about 0.2 ounces or 5 grams)

¼ cup chopped fresh mint leaves (about 0.2 ounces or 5 grams)

Extra virgin olive oil: I used Private Reserve Greek extra virgin olive oil

Vegetables: 1 large chopped onion, 1 to 2 green bell peppers, and 2 minced garlic cloves. These three ingredients (plus spices) creates a sofrito to start the chunky sauce.

Spices: coriander, cumin, paprika-- a trio of warm North African flavors. If you like spicy shakshuka (some call it eggs in purgatory), add a pinch of red pepper flakes or cayenne pepper.

Tomatoes (and alternatives): In this recipe, I use 6 chopped vine ripe tomatoes and about ½ cup of tomato sauce, this combination gives me the texture and flavor I'm looking for. It helps if your tomatoes are soft and almost overripe. You can also replace the fresh tomatoes with 1 28-ounce can of whole tomatoes or 6 cups of chopped tomatoes from a can with their juices.

Eggs: 6 large eggs (raw)

Garnish: This is totally optional, but for me a handful of fresh chopped parsley and mint just before serving adds freshness and a pop of color.

Directions

Heat 3 tbsp olive oil in a large cast iron skillet. Add the onions, green peppers, garlic, spices, pinch salt and pepper. Cook, stirring occasionally, until the vegetables have softened, about 5 minutes.

Add the tomatoes and tomato sauce. Cover and let simmer for about 15 minutes. Uncover and cook a bit longer to allow the mixture to reduce and thicken. Taste and adjust the seasoning to your liking.

Using a wooden spoon, make 6 indentations, or "wells," in the tomato mixture (make sure the indentations are spaced out). Gently crack an egg into each indention.

Reduce the heat, cover the skillet, and cook on low until the egg whites are set.

Uncover and add the fresh parsley and mint. You can add more black pepper or crushed red pepper, if you like. Serve with warm pita, challah bread, or your choice of crusty bread.

Moroccan Vegetable Tagine

A tagine is a conical cooking pot with a shallow base and tall, cone-shaped lid that is commonly used to make tagines, or stews. The name of the dish and the name of the meal cooking inside of it are the same. The benefit to cooking a tagine (the meal) in a tagine (the pot) is the pot seals in all of the flavorful ingredients that usually have a bit of moisture from sauce and vegetables, then that moisture goes up the sides of the lid and back down over the ingredients, creating a self-basting, flavor-enhancing cycle of deliciousness.

Ingredients

¼ cup Private Reserve extra virgin olive oil, more for later

2 medium yellow onions, peeled and chopped

8-10 garlic cloves, peeled and chopped

2 large carrots, peeled and chopped

2 large russet potatoes, peeled and cubed

1 large sweet potato, peeled and cubed

Salt

1 tbsp Harissa spice blend

1 tsp ground coriander

1 tsp ground cinnamon

½ tsp ground turmeric

2 cups canned whole peeled tomatoes

½ cup heaping chopped dried apricot

1 quart low-sodium vegetable broth (or broth of your choice)

2 cups cooked chickpeas

1 lemon, juice of

Handful fresh parsley leaves

Directions

In a large heavy pot or Dutch Oven, heat olive oil over medium heat until just shimmering. Add onions and increase heat to medium-high. Saute for 5 minutes, tossing regularly.

Add garlic and all the chopped veggies. Season with salt and spices. Toss to combine.

Cook for 5 to 7 minutes on medium-high heat, mixing regularly with a wooden spoon.

Add tomatoes, apricot and broth. Season again with just a small dash of salt.

Keep the heat on medium-high, and cook for 10 minutes. Then reduce heat, cover and simmer for another 20 to 25 minutes or until veggies are tender.

Stir in chickpeas and cook another 5 minutes on low heat.

Stir in lemon juice and fresh parsley. Taste and adjust seasoning, adding more salt or harissa spice blend to your liking.

Transfer to serving bowls and top each with a generous drizzle of Private Reserve extra virgin olive oil. Serve hot with your favorite bread, couscous, or rice. Enjoy!

Best Paleo Chili

A hearty bowl of chili is the perfect dinner for a blustery winter day. This one in particular is one of our favorites. It's spicy, super savory, and extra hearty. We can't get enough of it! Read on to learn exactly what makes this chili so special. It's packed with veggies. It's a common misconception that paleo dieters subsist solely on meat. Untrue! Veggies are an important part of any diet, and this chili makes sure you get the good stuff in! It's packed with celery, peppers, and onions, and could be adapted to make way for even more vegetables. Try stirring in some chopped cauliflower with the onions, or stir in kale near the end of cooking time and simmer until it's wilted. It's got all the classic chili flavors. Since fruits are tricky ingredients to navigate on paleo, it might come as a surprise that you can eat tomatoes. Because they're relatively low on the glycemic index they're totally safe to eat. Fire roasted tomatoes + lots of chili powder, cumin, and oregano = big chili flavor. Once you try chili topped with bacon, you're never going back. To offset all that salty, fatty goodness we've got bright cilantro, spicy jalapeño, and creamy avocado. It's all about balance. It's a meal-preppers dream. Chili, like many soups and stews, is better on day 2. This makes this chili the PERFECT food for meal prep— it gets better as the week goes on! Just keep your toppers separate, microwave the chili when you're ready to eat and top as desired.

Ingredients

3 slices bacon, cut into 1/2" strips

1/2 medium yellow onion, chopped

2 celery stalks, chopped

2 bell peppers, chopped

3 cloves garlic, minced

2 lb. lean ground beef

2 tbsp. chili powder

2 tsp. ground cumin

2 tsp. dried oregano

2 tbsp. smoked paprika

Kosher salt

Freshly ground black pepper

1 (28-oz.) can fire-roasted tomatoes

2 c. low-sodium chicken broth

Sliced jalapeños, for garnish

Sliced avocado, for garnish

freshly chopped cilantro, for garnish

Directions

In a large pot over medium heat, cook bacon. When bacon is crisp, remove from pot with a slotted spoon. Add onion, celery, and peppers to pot and cook until soft, 6 minutes. Add garlic and cook until fragrant, 1 minute more.

Push vegetables to one side of the pan and add beef. Cook, stirring occasionally, until no pink remains. Drain fat and return to heat.

Add chili powder, cumin, oregano, and paprika and season with salt and pepper. Stir to combine and cook 2 minutes more. Add tomatoes and broth and bring to a simmer. Let cook 10 to 15 more minutes, until chili has thickened slightly.

Ladle into bowls and top with reserved bacon, jalapeños, cilantro, and avocado.

Homemade Hummus

Hummus is an incredibly popular Middle Eastern dip and spread. It is typically made by blending chickpeas (garbanzo beans), tahini (ground sesame seeds), olive oil, lemon juice and garlic in a food processor. Not only is hummus delicious, but it is also versatile, packed with nutrients and has been linked to many impressive health and nutritional benefits

Ingredients

Chickpeas (3 cups). Chickpeas, also known as garbanzo beans, are the star ingredient in hummus. Canned or dry chickpeas? If you're wondering how to make hummus from scratch--the best, extra creamy, authentic stuff--you'll want to cook your own chickpeas from scratch (you'll give them a good soak overnight + boil in water until well-done. More on this later)

Garlic (1 or 2 cloves). Start with 1 clove and make sure it is finely minced. Tip: to tame its pungency, allow minced garlic to sit in a little bit of lemon juice for a few minutes.

Tahini (⅓ cup). Tahini is a rich, nutty and slightly bitter paste made from toasted sesame seeds. (You can find my go-to tahini paste here).

Fresh Lemon Juice (from 1 lemon). Fresh lemon juice is just the thing to add tang here.

Kosher Salt. Just a pinch of kosher salt to your liking. You can always add more. If you're interested in adding

Extra Virgin Olive Oil. A generous drizzle of quality extra virgin olive oil is the way to finish and serve this dip the authentic way. (You can find my go-to extra virgin olive oils at our online shop here)

Garnish. Not to be underestimated. My favorite way to garnish a bowl of hummus, once the EVOO has been poured nicely right in the middle, is a few pinches of tangy sumac (sometimes ground cumin is a good addition). If you have some extra cooked chickpeas, plant them right in the middle. For a pop of green, you can add a garnish of fresh parsley.

bowl of hummus with olive oil and chickpeas. A side of pita bread

Ingredients

3 cups cooked chickpeas, peeled (from 1 to 1 ¼ cup dry chickpeas or from quality canned chickpeas. See recipe notes for more instructions on cooking and peeling chickpeas)

1 to 2 garlic cloves, minced

3 to 4 ice cubes

⅓ cup (79 grams) tahini paste

½ tsp kosher salt

Juice of 1 lemon

Hot water (if needed)

Early Harvest Greek extra virgin olive oil

Sumac

Directions

Add chickpeas and minced garlic to the bowl of a
food processor. Puree until a smooth, powder-like
mixture forms.

While processor is running, add ice cubes, tahini,
salt, and lemon juice. Blend for about 4 minutes or

so. Check, and if the consistency is too thick still, run processor and slowly add a little hot water. Blend until you reach desired silky smooth consistency.

Spread in a serving bowl and add a generous drizzle of Early Harvest EVOO. Add a few chickpeas to the middle, if you like. Sprinkle sumac on top. Enjoy with warm pita wedges and your favorite veggies.

Tahini Sauce

Tahini is a super creamy, rich vegan paste made by finely grinding roasted sesame seeds until buttery smooth. I've heard some referring to tahini as a "nut butter" of sorts. It's important to remember though that seeds--sesame, sunflower, poppy, and pumpkin--come from plant families that are not closely related to nut-producing trees.

Ingredients

1-2 garlic cloves

½ tsp salt

¾ cup tahini paste

½ cup freshly squeezed lime juice (or lemon juice, if you prefer)

¼ cup cold water, more if needed

1 cup fresh chopped parsley leaves, stems removed first (optional)

Directions

Using a mortar and pestle, crush the garlic cloves with the salt into a paste (or mince the garlic and season with salt.)

Add the crushed garlic, tahini paste and lime juice to the bowl of a food processor and blend (it will be thick as it emulsifies.) Add a little bit of water and blend again until you reach the desired consistency.

Transfer the tahini to a serving bowl, and if you like stir in fresh chopped parsley. Enjoy!

Grilled Salmon Kabobs

These grilled Salmon and lemon Kabobs are too easy to make, loaded with omega 3s in every bite. It's seasoned with fresh herbs, lemon, and spices and grilled to perfection. It maintains your health as it contains only a low carb of 7 grams and is a high protein recipe. It's too delicious and is one of the perfect low carb high protein recipes for a quick snack.

Ingredients

2 tbsp chopped fresh oregano

2 tsp sesame seeds

1 tsp ground cumin

1/4 tsp crushed red pepper flakes

1-1/2 pounds skinless wild salmon fillet, cut into 1-inch pieces

2 lemons, very thinly sliced into rounds

olive oil cooking spray

1 tsp kosher salt

16 bamboo skewers soaked in water 1 hour

Directions

Heat the grill on medium heat and spray the grates with oil.

Mix oregano, sesame seeds, cumin, and red pepper flakes in a small bowl to combine; set spice mixture aside.

Beginning and ending with salmon, thread salmon and folded lemon slices onto 8 pairs of parallel skewers to make 8 kebabs total.

Spray the fish lightly with oil and season kosher salt and the reserved spice mixture.

Grill the fish, turning occasionally, until fish is opaque throughout, about 8 to 10 minutes total.

Chicken Broccoli Bake

These easy Chicken and Broccoli Casserole are a simple and delicious keto dinner that is ready in not more than 25 minutes. It is rich and healthy with amazing flavors and contains only 6 grams of total carbs. You are gonna crave more once you taste this recipe. It's too creamy, hearty, and cheesy and also is suitable for an easy one-pan meal.

Ingredients

1/4 cup butter, divided

12 ounces broccoli , coarsely chopped

2 cloves garlic, minced

1 cup heavy whipping cream

1 1/2 cups shredded mozzarella, divided

1/2 cup grated parmesan cheese

Salt and pepper

3 cups cooked chopped chicken (about 1 1/4 lbs)

Directions

Set a 10-inch ovenproof skillet over medium heat and add 2 tablespoons of the butter. Once melted, add the broccoli and sauté until bright green and just tender, about 4 minutes. Remove the broccoli to a bowl.

Melt the remaining butter in the pan and add the garlic, cooking until fragrant, about 1 minute. Add the cream and bring to a simmer, then cook until reduced by about half, 3 to 5 minutes.

Stir in 1/2 cup of the mozzarella and all of the Parmesan until melted. Season with salt and pepper to taste. Stir in the broccoli and the chicken and top with the remaining 1 cup of mozzarella cheese.

Preheat the broiler. Set the pan about 6 inches from the heat and broil until the cheese is beginning to brown, 2 to 5 minutes (depends on how intense your broiler is!).

Homemade Chicken Tikka Masala

Ingredients

for 5 servings

CHICKEN MARINADE

3 boneless, skinless chicken breasts

½ cup plain yogurt(125 g)

2 tablespoons lemon juice

6 cloves garlic, minced

1 tablespoon minced ginger

2 teaspoons salt

2 teaspoons ground cumin

2 teaspoons garam masala

2 teaspoons paprika

SAUCE

3 tablespoons oil

1 large onion, finely chopped

2 tablespoons minced ginger

8 cloves garlic, minced

2 teaspoons ground cumin

2 teaspoons ground turmeric

2 teaspoons ground coriander

2 teaspoons paprika

2 teaspoons chili powder

2 teaspoons garam masala

1 tablespoon tomato puree

3 ½ cups tomato sauce(800 g)

1 ¼ cups water(300 mL)

1 cup heavy cream(250 mL)

¼ cup fresh cilantro(10 g), for garnish

cooked rice, for serving

naan bread, for serving

SPECIAL EQUIPMENT

Bamboo or wooden skewer

Directions

Slice the chicken into bite-sized chunks. Combine the cubed chicken with the yogurt, lemon juice, garlic, ginger, salt, cumin, garam masala, and paprika and stir until well-coated.

Cover and refrigerate for at least 1 hour, or overnight.

Preheat the oven to 500°F (260°C). Line a high-sided baking pan or roasting tray with parchment paper.

Place the marinated chicken pieces on bamboo or wooden skewers, then set them over the prepared baking pan, making sure there is space underneath the chicken to help distribute the heat more evenly.

Bake for about 15 minutes, until slightly dark brown on the edges.

Make the sauce: Heat the oil in a large pot over medium heat, then sauté the onions, ginger, and garlic until tender but not browned. Add the cumin, turmeric, coriander, paprika, chili powder, and garam masala and stir constantly for about 30 seconds, until the spices are fragrant. Stir in the tomato puree, tomato sauce, and 1 ¼ cups of water, then bring to a boil and cook for about 5 minutes. Pour in the cream.

Remove the chicken from the skewers and add to the sauce, cooking for another 1-2 minutes. Garnish with cilantro and serve over rice or alongside naan bread.

Enjoy!

Ginger Turmeric Chicken Soup

Ingredients

for 6 servings

4 cups water(1 L)

1 ½ lb Simple Truth® Chicken Breasts(655 g)

2 bay leaves

1 teaspoon whole black peppercorn

1 teaspoon kosher salt, plus more to taste

1 ½ tablespoons olive oil

1 small yellow onion, diced

2 medium carrots, sliced 1/4 (6 mm) think on the bias

1 ¾ cups shiitake mushroom(110 g), sliced

2 cloves garlic, minced

5 teaspoons grated fresh ginger

1 ½ teaspoons ground ginger

1 teaspoon ground turmeric

2 sprigs fresh rosemary

1 cup dinosaur kale(40 g)

8 cups chicken stock(1.6 L)

¼ lb angel hair pasta(105 g), broken crosswise into thirds

freshly ground black pepper, to taste

Directions

In a medium pot, bring the water to a simmer, about 5 minutes. Add the Simple Truth® Chicken Breasts, bay leaves, whole black peppercorns, and salt. Cook until the internal temperature of the chicken reaches 165°F (75°C), about 15 minutes. Remove the chicken from the poaching liquid and transfer to a cutting board. Let cool enough to handle, then dice into ¾" pieces.

In a large pot, heat the olive oil over medium-low heat. Add the onion and sauté until translucent, about 2 minutes. Add the carrots and mushrooms, and cook until softened, about 3 minutes. Add the garlic and fresh ginger, and cook until fragrant, 30–45 seconds. Add the ground ginger, turmeric, rosemary, and kale. Stir to combine for 30 seconds, then pour in the chicken stock. Bring to a simmer and cook for 10–15 minutes.

Increase the heat to medium-high to bring the soup to a boil, then add the angel hair pasta and diced Simple Truth® Chicken Breasts. Cook according to the package instructions until the pasta is tender. Season with salt and pepper to taste.

Serve warm.

Enjoy!

Tofu Tikka Masala

Ingredients

for 4 servings

MARINADE

14 oz extra firm tofu(395 g)

1 lemon

1 cup yogurt(245 g)

6 cloves garlic, minced

1 tablespoon ginger, minced

1 teaspoon salt

2 teaspoons cumin

2 teaspoons garam masala

2 teaspoons paprika

SAUCE

3 tablespoons oil

1 large onion, finely chopped

2 tablespoons ginger, minced

8 cloves garlic, minced

2 teaspoons cumin

2 teaspoons turmeric

2 teaspoons coriander powder

2 teaspoons paprika

2 teaspoons chili powder

2 teaspoons garam masala

3 ½ cups tomato sauce(800 g), or crushed tomatoes

1 ¼ cups water(300 mL)

1 cup heavy cream(250 mL), or dairy substitute of your choice

fresh coriander, chopped, to garnish

rice, to serve

naan bread, to serve

Directions

Remove tofu from packaging and drain.

Place tofu on a couple of paper towels and find a heavy object to place on top of tofu, leave it there for 20 minutes.

Slice the tofu into bite-sized pieces.

Combine the marinade ingredients in a bowl then add the tofu.

Mix until evenly coated. Cover and refrigerate for at least 1 hour.

Preheat oven to 425°F (220°C)

Place the marinated tofu pieces on bamboo skewers, then place them over a baking tray lined with parchment paper. Make sure there is space underneath the tofu to help distribute the heat more evenly.

Bake for about 15 minutes, until slightly dark brown on the edges.

Heat oil in a large pot over medium heat, and sauté the onions, ginger, and garlic until tender but not browned.

Add the spices for about 30 seconds to release their aromatics and flavor, stirring constantly.

Add the tomato sauce and water, then bring to a boil and cook for about 5 minutes.

Pour in the cream and mix in the tofu, cooking for another 1-2 minutes.

Serve with rice and naan bread.

Enjoy!

Channa Masala

Ingredients

for 4 servings

1 tablespoon olive oil

1 large yellow onion, diced

2 cloves garlic, minced

1 tablespoon grated fresh ginger

1 green chile, or jalapeño, seeded and finely chopped

2 tablespoons garam masala

1 teaspoon turmeric

1 teaspoon kosher salt

1 teaspoon freshly ground black pepper

2 cups diced tomatoes(400 g)

30 oz chickpeas(425 g), drained and rinsed

½ cup water(120 mL)

½ lemon, juiced

¼ cup chopped fresh cilantro(10 g), chopped

cooked basmati rice, for serving (optional)

naan bread, for serving (optional)

Directions

Heat the olive oil in a large stockpot or Dutch oven over medium-high heat.

Add the onion and cook until translucent and beginning to brown, 3–5 minutes.

Add the garlic, ginger, and green chile and continue to cook over medium heat until the garlic is fragrant and the chile is tender, 3–4 minutes.

Add the garam masala, turmeric, salt, and black pepper, then continue to cook for 1–2 minutes.

Add the tomatoes, chickpeas, and water. Stir to incorporate, using the spoon to scrape up any browned bits from the bottom and sides of the pot. As the tomatoes break down, the mixture should take on the consistency of a thick stew. Add more water if needed before bringing everything to a simmer, then cover with the lid and cook, stirring occasionally, for 15 minutes.

Remove the lid, reduce the heat to low, and stir in the lemon juice and cilantro. Cook for 1–2 minutes, until the cilantro has wilted and turned bright green.

Serve over basmati rice or with a side of naan.

Enjoy!

Chili Chicken-stuffed Parathas

Ingredients

for 5 servings

1 tablespoon oil

1 tablespoon garlic ginger paste

1 red chili, diced

1 onion, diced

1 tomato, chopped

1 teaspoon chili powder

1 teaspoon turmeric

1 tablespoon garam masala

1 teaspoon salt

1 teaspoon pepper

3 ¼ cups chicken(400 g), cooked and shredded

1 bunch fresh coriander, small bunch, chopped

10 parathas, defrosted

Directions

Heat the oil in a large saucepan over a medium heat.

Fry the garlic and ginger paste for a couple of minutes.

Stir in the chili and onion and fry for about 5 minutes, until soft.

Add the tomato, followed by the chili powder, turmeric, garam masala, salt, and pepper.

Fry for another few minutes stirring continuously.

Stir in the chicken and coriander and mix until evenly coated.

Set the pan aside.

In a smaller pan over medium heat, place on a paratha. Spoon on some of the chicken mix and place another paratha on top.

Carefully seal the sides with your fingers, being careful not to touch the pan.

Cook for a few minutes on each side until crisp and golden brown.

Slice the parathas in half and serve with chutneys, raitas, or any other dips of your choice.

Enjoy!

Kerala-Style Prawn Curry

Ingredients

for 4 servings

1 tablespoon cooking oil

1 teaspoon fenugreek

½ teaspoon turmeric

¼ teaspoon asafoetida

1 teaspoon mustard seed

12 leaves dried curry

2 lb fresh king prawn(1 kg)

1 cup coconut milk(200 mL)

¼ cup water(50 mL)

salt, to season

pepper, to season

1 lime, juiced

PASTE

1 onion, chopped

1 red chili

⅔cup ginger(30 g)

4 cloves garlic

Directions

In a food processor, blitz the onion, chili, ginger and garlic together to make a paste. Set aside.

In a large pan, heat the oil over a medium heat.

Add the fenugreek, turmeric, asafoetida, mustard seeds, and curry leaves to the pan, and fry for a couple of minutes.

Add the paste and continue to cook for 2-3 minutes.

Add the prawns and water. Cook until they start to turn pink.

Pour in the coconut milk, salt, pepper, and lime juice, and cook for another few minutes.

Serve with parathas, naan bread, and rice.

Enjoy!

Anti-Inflammatory Golden Milk

Ingredients

for 2 servings

2 cups almond milk(480 mL), or other non-dairy milk

1 tablespoon ground turmeric

¼ teaspoon ground ginger

4 black peppercorns

1 stick cinnamon

1 star anise

1 pinch whole clove

1 teaspoon agave, or sweetener of your choice, optional

Directions

Add the almond milk to a small pot over medium heat.

Add the turmeric, ginger, peppercorns, cinnamon stick, star anise, and cloves. Whisk to combine.

Heat the milk for 4-5 minutes, until steaming, but do not let it come to a boil.

Serve warm or over ice and sweeten to taste.

Enjoy!

Anti-Inflammatory Aid Wellness Shot

Ingredients

for 4 shots

2 oranges, juiced

2 lemons, juiced

1 inch piece fresh turmeric, peeled

⅛ teaspoon black pepper

⅛ teaspoon cayenne

Directions

Combine the orange juice, lemon juice, turmeric, pepper, and cayenne in a blender and blend until smooth.

Divide among 4 shot glasses.

Enjoy

CHAPTER NINE

JUST ONE FINAL THING TO ADDRESS BEFORE YOU GO!

Management approaches for lipoedema and lymphoedema differ significantly due to their distinct nature and underlying causes. While both conditions lack a definitive cure, various treatments exist to mitigate their impact on individuals' lives.

Lymphoedema, characterized by the accumulation of lymphatic fluid, is commonly managed through a multifaceted approach. This typically involves incorporating light exercise into daily routines, as movement can stimulate lymphatic flow and reduce swelling. Additionally, pneumatic compression devices, specialized bandages, and manual lymphatic drainage techniques administered by trained professionals are utilized to alleviate symptoms and promote fluid drainage. In severe cases where conservative measures prove insufficient, surgical intervention may be considered to excise excess tissue and alleviate persistent swelling.

On the other hand, lipoedema, characterized by abnormal fat accumulation, requires a tailored management strategy. While exercise and lifestyle modifications are often recommended to promote overall health and weight management, traditional weight loss methods may not effectively target lipoedema fat deposits. As a result, specialized treatments such as manual lymphatic drainage, compression therapy, and specific dietary interventions may be employed to manage symptoms and improve quality of life. In some instances, liposuction surgery performed by skilled surgeons trained in lipoedema management may be considered to remove excess fat deposits and alleviate discomfort.

Overall, the management of lipoedema and lymphoedema necessitates a comprehensive and individualized approach that addresses the unique characteristics and challenges of each condition. Collaborating closely with healthcare professionals, including physicians, physiotherapists, and lymphedema therapists, can help individuals develop personalized treatment plans tailored to their specific needs and goals. By combining various therapeutic modalities and lifestyle adjustments, individuals can effectively manage their symptoms and optimize their overall well-being despite the chronic nature of these conditions.